The Suddenly Successful Student

A Guide to Overcoming Learning & Behavior Problems

How Behavioral Optometry Helps

Hazel Dawkins
Dr. Ellis Edelman • Dr. Constantine Forkiotis

i

Copyright © 1990 The Writing Team
Printed in the United States of America

Library of Congress Cataloging-in-Publication Data
Dawkins, Hazel H. Richmond, 1937-
    The Suddenly Successful Student:
    A Guide to Overcoming
    Learning and Behavior Problems,
    How Behavioral Optometry Helps / Hazel
Richmond Dawkins, Ellis Edelman, Constantine Forkiotis.

Third edition — Originally published: Lititz, Pa. : Sutter
House, copyright 1986.
    Edelman's name appears first on the earlier edition.
Includes bibliographical references and index.

    Cover design and art and internal design by
        Colin Dawkins II and Kyo Takahashi

ISBN 0-943599-15-6: $8.50

1. Vision disorders in children—Handbooks, manuals, etc.
2. Children—Medical examinations—Handbooks, manuals,
etc.
I. Edelman, Ellis S., 1924- .
II. Forkiotis, Constantine, 1923- .
III. Title
RE48.2.C5E34 1990
618.92'0977-dc20   90-7828
                                        CIP

Contents

Preface

Doctors Ellis Edelman and Constantine Forkiotis have specialized in behavioral optometry for many years, painstakingly accumulating the knowledge that has gone into this handbook. To this, Hazel Richmond Dawkins has brought her personal experience. When she was seven years of age, she had an operation to "straighten" an in-turning eye. Within months, the eye was turning out. For the next forty years, Hazel was functionally blind in that eye. During those years, in England, France, Switzerland and America, she was told nothing could be done, although the eye was "healthy."

Imagine, then, her amazement when she was referred to Dr. Ellis Edelman, a Pennsylvania behavioral optometrist, and learned that her "blindness" was the result of the brain shutting down input from that eye because it didn't fuse with the input from her other eye. She discovered there was a distinct possibility she could learn to straighten her eye without surgery, and perhaps recover some of the lost sight and vision. Behavioral optometry offered vision therapy, and in the following months the hoped-for changes did materialize.

In rapid succession, Hazel's husband and three of their five children consulted with Dr. Edelman and were helped to an extraordinary degree. It was at this point that Hazel realized the need for information to be written for general readers and enlisted the collaboration of Drs. Edelman and Forkiotis.

Others, particularly the following, have given their support and advice, for which the authors thank them: Drs. Elliott Forrest, Irwin Suchoff, Nathan Flax, Harold Solan and Beth Bazin of New York's SUNY; Dr. David Friedel, Tucson; Dr. Lynn Hellerstein, Denver; Dr. Beth Ballinger, Newport Beach; Charlotte A. Rancilio of AOA; Dr. Martin Kane of

COVD; Dr. Richard Apell and Mary Megargee of the Gesell Institute of Human Development; Dr. Charles Margach of Southern California College of Optometry; Dr. Gerry Getman of Maryland and Robert Williams and the staff at the OEP Foundation.

Hazel Richmond Dawkins
Ellis Edelman
Constantine Forkiotis

Fact Sheet

Behavioral (also described as functional or developmental) optometry is a rapidly growing therapy in the field of optometry.

Roughly 30 percent of the individuals in any school, college or office have difficulties with learning, work and health that have nothing to do with their natural intelligence. Their problem lies with their vision.

Youngsters with vision problems are often labeled slow learner, problem child, learning disabled, dyslexic and delinquent. Most vision imbalances are triggered or aggravated by stress or the visual demands of work or computer use.

Sight and vision are not the same, there is a critical difference between them: Sight is the ability of the eyes to focus, one of many different skills that make up vision. When skills such as converging, fixation and teaming integrate efficiently with the brain's visual cortex so you understand what you see, the result is vision.

Sight is the ability to *see*, to look at an object and have it in focus. When we use our *vision*, the brain organizes the information *seen* and gives it meaning, often by relating it to our other senses and past experience. Vision is the ability to understand what is seen.

Vision develops in a sequence of predictable stages. Therefore, it is trainable.

Vision problems may trigger or aggravate health, learning or behavior problems. When behavioral optometry brings balance to vision, often the health, learning or behavior problems may be helped and will respond to traditional therapies such as remedial education or counseling which might not have been effective before optometric vision therapy.

The concepts, practices and lens use of this optometric therapy are different from general optometry and ophthalmology. In general, most lenses prescribed by general optometrists and ophthalmologists are compensating. Behavioral optometry uses lenses in ways that are remedial, developmental and preventive.

Remedial lenses are for a specific problem, such as an inability to sustain focusing, until that ability is adequate.

Developmental lenses are to support and nurture an immature vision system while helping it develop normally and cope with visual stress.

Preventive lenses are to prevent a problem in the vision system from starting in those individuals diagnosed "at risk."

The ability to see and correctly interpret what is seen does not appear automatically at birth. It develops during the first twelve years of life and is shaped by health, one's experiences and the environment.

Optometrists—The O.D. degree stands for Doctor of Optometry. It is earned after a minimum of seven years of college and graduate education. Optometry's areas of specialization range from contact lenses to pediatric vision. One of the most innovative is vision therapy, for which postdoctoral training is needed.

General optometrists offer routine eye health care and refraction (the clinical measurement of the eye to determine the need for lenses). Their extensive education has prepared general optometrists to detect not only ocular diseases but signs of certain health problems such as hypertension, diabetes and arteriosclerosis.

Behavioral (developmental or functional) optometrists practice vision therapy, sometimes in addition to general optometry, sometimes exclusively. In contrast to general optometrists and ophthalmologists, who usually believe that visual problems stem from random or genetic biological variations, behavioralists believe that visual problems are also triggered by environmental factors which may be developmental or stress-induced.

Ophthalmologists are doctors of medicine (M.Ds.) whose postgraduate training is in diseases of the eye.

Opticians are technicians who produce and/or dispense the optical lenses, glasses or other equipment prescribed by optometrists and ophthalmologists.

Optometric vision therapy works on the visual perceptual system (the eye, oculomotor muscles and pathways, the optic nerve and optic tract and that part of the brain used in vision processing). Warps or imbalances at any point in this complex system will lead to faulty processing of visual information. This in turn may trigger a host of behavior, learning, work and health problems.

Age is not a deterrent to the benefits of optometric vision therapy. Infants of two months can be helped, adults in their seventies can benefit.

Health insurance companies such as Aetna Life & Casualty Company and Blue Cross/Blue Shield have plans that cover optometric vision therapy—and have done so for years.

1

A Parents' and Teachers' Guide to Vision Problems

About ten million children under the age of twelve in the United States have vision problems that make it hard for them to cope with home and school.

That's the bad news. It comes from the American Optometric Association (AOA), the nation's leading professional organization devoted to the problems of vision and vision care. The AOA makes an important distinction between vision and sight. "Rarely do these *vision* conditions threaten a child's *sight*." However, "They do...often prevent a child's development into a normal, contributing adult...by interfering with learning; inhibiting participation in sports...and creating frustration that leads to misbehavior, dropping out of school and even juvenile delinquency."

The Association's warning is clear. It is well-documented that youngsters with vision problems usually have difficulties with learning in school. They often have trouble dealing with family and fiends. They may become so frustrated by their problems that they retreat into rebellion. they can become dropouts. Suicides. Or menaces to society.

These youngsters are often given gaudy labels: juvenile delinquent, problem child, slow learner, dyslexic, learning- disabled. The sad truth is that giving children with vision problems such labels is like jailing them for crimes which they just didn't commit.

The good news is this: In almost every case of a child with a vision problem there is a relatively simple solution. It can be supplied by a doctor of optometry who specializes in "behavioral optometry."

The trick is: Recognizing the child with the problem and getting the child to the correct practitioner. Parents, teachers, all of us need to know the symptoms of vision problems. We need to know there is a difference between sight and vision.

"Sight" is the ability of the eyes to focus, one of many different skills which make up vision. "Vision" is something all-embracing. When skills such as converging, fixation and teaming integrate efficiently with the brain's visual cortex so that you understand what you see, the result is "Vision."

We also need to know that the professionals who treat these broad-based vision problems are doctors of optometry who specialize in a particular branch of optometry, behavioral optometry, sometimes called functional or developmental.

Their Eyesight May Be Good
But Their Vision May Be Terrible

As a parent or a teacher, you must be able to make this distinction. Most children have healthy eyes. They can score an easy 20/20 on the eyecharts. Even if one eye is a little near- or farsighted and the other is not. That is "sight."

"Vision," however, is another thing. If, for instance, one eye is a little farsighted and the other eye is a little nearsighted, they are not able to work together as a team. The message they send to the brain is confusing. One eye delivers one message to the brain,the other eye delivers another.

To a child this is like being told by the father to do one thing and by the mother to do another. The messages are contradictory. So the child is faced with a dilemma. Which parent—which eye message—does the youngster heed?

When a child's brain is confused by contradictory messages from the eyes, the body becomes a battleground. Under the most extreme circumstances, the brain makes one of several choices. The two discussed here are radical decisions:

1. The brain stops accepting messages from one eye;
2. The brain alternates reception from one eye to the other, this slows understanding and creates confusion.

This failure of the eyes to work together as a team is called, appropriately enough, "lack of teaming." A teacher can expect to find symptoms of it in about 5 percent of a classroom's students. Once discovered, the child should be examined by a doctor of optometry who specializes in behavioral optometric vision care.

Lack of teaming is only one of a number of vision problems that can affect learning and behavior. Spotting the symptoms of such vision problems is a challenge for parents and teachers.

2

Does This Remind You of Someone You Know?

James   He's in third grade. He's obviously bright. But Jimmy can't read as well as his brother in first grade.

Sharon   She's a brat, according to her family. Won't cooperate. Won't do as she's asked. Has temper tantrums. Cries a lot. She's ten years old.

Max   He's fifteen. He's surly, unfriendly. Doesn't communicate with family or schoolmates. He's on his way to being a dropout. Yet he's not dumb because he can repeat every commercial he's ever heard on television.

Kevin   He's seventeen, tall, strong and handsome. Yet he's never been able to be active in any team sport. He gets violently car sick, can't watch television or do homework without getting a headache.

| Sally | Everybody knows she's brilliant because she reads incessantly, anything and everything. But she does poorly in school and tests show this thirteen-year-old does not understand a lot of what she reads. That came as a surprise to her parents. |

Every teacher and many parents will recognize such behavior problems. Roughly 10 percent of the students in any classroom will exhibit these or similar difficulties. The youngsters involved will come under the scrutiny of family, teachers, therapists, psychologists and doctors (depending on the symptoms). And these well-meaning people will suggest all kinds of reasons for such problems: lazy, not trying, hyperactive, emotionally disturbed, learning disabled, delinquent, brain damaged, dyslexic.

Yet all the individuals mentioned here—from James to Sally—are bright kids who are being victimized by problems in their vision systems. One of the most fearful oversights in medicine, education and psychology today is the neglect of children's vision systems. We routinely test for "eyesight" but rarely for "vision imbalances." And, as a result, we allow some of our best and brightest to go down the drain. Every parent and every teacher should know that this *doesn't have to happen.* A classic example is Luci Baines Johnson.

Luci Baines Johnson.

When she was a teenager and her father was vice-president of the United States, Luci Johnson was having serious problems with her schoolwork. Her parents, both overachievers, were deeply worried and somewhat embarrassed. Despite their wealth, despite their access to all kinds of learned advice, despite having explored every possible avenue, nothing they had tried had helped.

Then Dr. Janet Travell, President John F. Kennedy's personal physician, suggested that Luci's vision might be at the center of the problem. Luci's parents responded that her eyes had been checked and she had 20/20 sight. Dr. Travell pointed out that Luci's *vision* had not been checked.

As a result, Luci was sent to Dr. Robert Kraskin, a Washington optometrist who specializes in behavioral optometric vision care. A small miracle happened, from Luci's point of view. Once she had completed a program of behavioral optometric care with Dr. Kraskin, she went from academic probation to honor roll. Not only did her schoolwork improve dramatically, she also began to be involved in sports from which her vision imbalance had previously barred her.

The change took time. Before vision care, Luci had experienced headaches and nausea when trying to deal with her schoolwork. But gradually, as her vision system came into better balance, Luci found that her ability to learn grew stronger. Like Luci Johnson, thousands of children and adults who've completed programs of optometric vision care have been able to improve learning and behavior and rid themselves of chronic health problems. Thousands more could benefit if they knew of this therapy and the optometric specialists who practice this preventive health care.

Psychiatry Expands Its Horizons

A study paper, "Visual Perceptual Dysfunction in Psychiatric Patients," by Frederic Flach, M.D., and Melvin Kaplan, O.D.,appeared in *Contemporary Psychiatry* of July-August 1983. More than half (66 percent) of the people in the seven-year study had"significant impairments in visual-perceptual function." In their conclusion, the authors wrote that "it would seem that there is definitely a relationship between certain psychiatric disorders and visual-perceptual dysfunction, particularly among patients diagnosed as having schizophrenic disorders, recurrent unipolar depression and alcoholism. Chronicity of illness (in excess of six months) and social withdrawal or occupational difficulties seem to be most marked among such patients.

"Although the exact nature of the relationship between dysfunction and psychopathology remains unclear, the fact that the presence or absence of such dysfunctions can be so easily determined should make us consider visual-perceptual analysis as a routine procedure in the evaluation of all psychiatric patients. Moreover, by means of visual training, the ability of such patients to function may often be substantially enhanced."

The authors had embarked on their research as the result of a poignant personal situation. Dr. Kaplan, a behavioral optometrist in Tarrytown, New York, had helped Dr. Flach's daughter with optometric vision therapy. A practitioner of this therapy since the 1960s, Dr. Kaplan is an instructor with the Department of Psychology at Mercy College, Dobbs Ferry, New York, and a member of the New York State Board of Examiners in Visual Training. Frederic Flach, M.D., has practiced psychiatry since the 1960s in New York City. He is an adjunct associate professor of psychiatry at the New York Hospital-Cornell Medical Center and Attending Psychiatrist at the Payne Whitney Clinic and St. Vincent's Hospital and Medical Center, New York. Both Dr. Kaplan and Dr. Flach have published in scientific journals.

When Dr. Flach took his daughter Rickie to Dr. Kaplan, Rickie was twenty-four. She had spent almost a decade in and out of psychiatric hospitals. Nothing, from drugs to therapy, had helped. Dr. Kaplan's examination of Rickie's vision system revealed a high level of spatial orientation dysfunction (difficulty knowing the accurate position of anything at which she looked). Dr. Kaplan combined optometric vision therapy and the constant use of lenses. A positive change was not long in coming. By the end of the first six weeks, Rickie's posture and dress had improved. By the end of the first twelve weeks, she was able to pass the test for a driving license and begin to drive a car. Within six months the young woman was discharged from hospital. She was able to attend college. Her life became thoroughly normal. In the years that followed, Rickie has not shown any symptoms of abnormal behavior or the schizophrenia that had haunted her. College, a job, marriage, motherhood, all these were made possible for Rickie to accomplish, once her vision system was brought into balance.

Note: Optometric vision therapy will not rid us of schizophrenia, depression, alcoholism, learning disabilities or the myriad problems that plague us. When such situations are vision-related, however, and vision is treated with optometric vision therapy, a firm foundation for overcoming such problems is established.

3

How You May Spot a Vision Imbalance

The kind of learning, behavior and health difficulties we are talking about probably will not be uncovered in the typical school eyechart examination or by an examination that is limited to checking eye health and eyesight. A thorough vision examination by a doctor of optometry who practices behavioral optometric vision care is wise.

Directly Observable

- Crossed or turned eyes

- Reddened, watering, burning or itching eyes; encrusted eyelids, frequent sties

- Turning or tilting head to use one eye only; or closing or covering one eye

- Placing head close to book or desk when reading or writing

- Frowning or scowling while reading, writing or doing chalkboard work

- Excessive blinking or rubbing of eyes

- Losing place while reading and using finger or marker to guide eyes

- Spidery, excessively sloppy or hard-to-read handwriting; writing that becomes smaller and crowded or inconsistent in size

Related to Behavior

- Short attention span for the child's age

- Nervousness, irritability, restlessness or unusual fatigue after visual concentration

- Displaying evidence of developmental or emotional immaturity

- Low frustration level; withdrawn, has difficulty getting along with other children

- Headaches, nausea and dizziness

- Complaints of blurring of vision or of double vision at any time

Related to Classroom Work

- Saying words aloud or lip reading

- Difficulty remembering what is read

- Omitting, repeating and miscalling words or confusion of similar words

- Persistent word reversals after the second grade

- Difficulty remembering, identifying and reproducing basic geometric forms

- Difficulty following verbal instructions

- Poor eye-hand coordination when copying from chalkboard, throwing or catching a ball, buttoning clothing, tying shoes.

If you notice such symptoms—and they can be subtle—you will be doing the child a lifetime service by calling on the expertise of a behavioral optometrist. They are usually the specialists equipped to diagnose and treat vision-related problems. Such imbalances of the vision system cannot always be corrected by the commonly prescribed eyeglasses or contact lenses. But optometric vision care, either lenses alone or in combination with therapy, can be effective in helping youngsters acquire vital vision skills.

All Children Need These Visual Skills
Not All Children Have Them

Many different visual skills are involved in a child's learning to cope with living in the complicated worlds of family and school. Young children must learn to understand what's going on around them in order to understand where they fit into things. Clear sight is not enough. Understanding, perception, is the key, and vision plays a major part in understanding. Children must first learn to read so that, later, they can read to learn. Similarly, the visual skills listed below are needed if youngsters are to succeed in school and in life.

1. Clearness of vision (acuity)
This is the ability to see clearly at near and far distances. (Clarity at distance is about the only skill that the usual eyechart examination tests, the Snellen eyechart exam that tells you that you have 20/20 acuity or you don't.)

Generally, children who have poor distance acuity are nearsighted—that is, do well at reading, less well at sports. The farsighted child tends to have more difficulty reading but, often, does better at sports than the nearsighted youngster.

2. Eye movement skills (fixation ability)

This is the ability to point the eyes accurately at an object and to keep the eyes on target whether the object is moving or stationary. Without these skills, you can't clearly follow a moving object, such as a ball in flight. You can't move your eyes smoothly across a line of text on a page. A child can't shift the eyes from a close object to a far one, such as from a notebook to a chalkboard in class.

3. Eye focusing skills (accommodation)

This is the ability to adjust the focus of the eyes as the distance from the object varies. Copying from the chalkboard, for instance, requires constant shifting of focus from far to near and back again. Most children are capable of a large amount of change of focus but fine, accurate control breaks down more easily under stress. Excellent eye focusing is a skill common to superior athletes.

4. Eye aiming skills (converging and diverging)

This is the ability to turn the eyes inward or outward in looking from objects close up to objects far away and back again. These skills must be closely coordinated with eye focusing skills. Inadequacies in these areas seriously hamper reading ability and athletic performance. Fortunately, these are skills that normally can be enhanced through optometric vision care.

5. Eye teaming skills (binocular fusion)

This is the ability to coordinate and align the eyes precisely so that the brain can fuse the input it receives from each eye. Even a slight misalignment can cause double vision, which, in turn, the brain may try to eliminate by suppressing the use of one eye. In one way or another, the brain will react in a disturbed and defensive manner to confusing signals from the eyes.

6. Eye-hand coordination

This is the ability of the vision system (eye-brain connection) to coordinate the information received through the eyes in order to monitor and direct the hands. This skill is important for learning to write (poor handwriting is often related to poor eye-hand coordination). It is essential to good performance in most sports.

7. Visual form perception

This is the ability to organize images on the printed page into letters and/or words. It is one of the most important skills used in learning to read and is developed through both experience and practice. It can be taught or improved.

What About Adults?

In the words of one expert, Allan Cott, M.D., a psychiatrist and best-selling author whose practice is in New York City, "Age is not a factor in the development of visual performance skills; such skills can be developed at any age." Dr. Cott adds that when learning, health and behavior problems are vision-related, optometric vision therapy can help the individual make changes and improvements to the vision system. This in turn will provide the individual with a firm foundation for beneficial change in other areas.

4

What Causes
Vision Problems?

M ost preschool children have good vision. Nevertheless, a small percentage of preschoolers have existing vision system problems. These can come from illnesses like measles or influenza. High fever, eye or head injury or pregnancy complications may also be factors. The fact is the majority of vision problems go unrecognized until the pressures of schoolwork and study begin to overload the vision system. The sudden impact of "nearpoint" work (reading, writing, drawing, doing numbers, using a computer) causes changes. A tendency to nearsightedness or farsightedness will become more pronounced. An eye may begin to cross or drift. Sight may become blurred or the child may begin to see double.

Most vision imbalances are triggered or aggravated by stress—often by the visual demands of schoolwork or by computer use.

This is a complication for parents and teachers because changes in children's vision usually happen so gradually that few children are aware of them. They assume that everyone sees the same way they do. This can be wildly misleading to the adults in their lives because children may have blurred sight or be seeing double and it will never occur to them to describe the condition.

That's why parents and teachers have to be alert to all the possible vision problems.

The Basic Conditions of Risk

Eye disease

The American Optometric Association (AOA) tells us that school-age children rarely have serious eye disease. But, AOA explains, there are two types of minor eye infections—blepharitis and sties—that may be indications of imbalances in the vision system. (Blepharitis is an inflammation of the eyelids, which can sometimes be identified by yellowish crusts at the base of the eyelashes.)

Both conditions, which are the results of stress caused by vision imbalances, call for a thorough examination of the complete vision system by a behavioral, functional or developmental optometrist.

Nearsightedness

What the eye doctor calls "myopia" is commonly called nearsightedness. The AOA tells us that "nearsightedness is the only refractive vision condition that increases significantly in incidence throughout the school years." You can expect to find it in about 3 percent of children between five and nine years of age. It increases in incidence to about 8 percent among children ten to twelve. And this rises along with the years of school experience to about 16 percent among teenagers. It's something to be on the lookout for.

Nearsighted individuals can see clearly up close but not at a distance. Watch students for these signs:

- A tendency to hold their books closer to their eyes than is normal;

- Bending their heads down close to the page when they write;

- Twisting their faces into a squint when they are trying to see the chalkboard.

Myopia—Preventive Treatment

The quick fix most often used for nearsightedness is prescription lenses. Lenses can compensate for and provide good visual acuity. The problem is that these "compensating" lenses usually need periodic changing and strengthening because myopia is usually progressive.

A more specialized and, in the long run, a more rewarding approach to nearsightedness is the preventive treatment of optometric vision therapy. This care takes the form of "learning" lenses (in contrast to "compensating" lenses) and vision therapy. Similarly, these and other special methodologies are also used to slow or stop the progression of nearsightedness (myopia control).

Nature designed human eyes primarily for sharp, clear seeing at a distance, the eyes of the hunter, the farmer, the sailor at sea. Our eyes were not designed for the endless stresses put upon them by modern living with our books, television viewing and computer screens, even high-speed travel.

Today, doctors of optometry who practice vision therapy can often prevent, reduce or control the myopia caused by environmental stresses by prescribing "learning" lenses. This type of lens has a mild prescription that reduces the amount of stress on the vision system. Usually, such learning lenses are necessary only for reading and close work.

Farsightedness

This is technically known as "hyperopia." The AOA tells us that most school-age children are farsighted—as nature intended them to be. They can usually see well at both distance and near; but there is a drawback. In most cases, farsighted children have to exert extra effort to bring their vision into sharp, clear focus for both far and near seeing.

For most such children, this presents no problem. But about 6 percent of children aged five to twelve have high degrees of farsightedness and need help to relieve the tension of focusing, especially when using their eyes for close work.

Again, most routine school eyechart examinations will not catch such problems. It's up to the parents and teachers to recognize the signs. Symptoms of hyperopia include:

- Difficulty in concentrating and maintaining a clear focus when reading or doing close work;

- Eye or body tension when doing such work;

- Muscle fatigue, headaches, nausea, aching or burning eyes after doing close work;

- Poor reading ability;

- Irritability or nervousness after sustained close-work concentration.

Astigmatism

This is the development of unequal curvature of the cornea. Thus, the light gathered in by the eye is not focused properly. The end result is blurred sight. The

AOA notes that only about 3 percent of school-age children have significant amounts of astigmatism; however, this represents an increase from 2 percent for preschoolers. The symptoms of astigmatism are similar to those for other vision disorders and they call for the same action: a thorough vision examination by an optometrist who practices behavioral, developmental or functional optometry.

Crossed Eyes and Lazy Eyes

Crossed eyes and lazy eyes are two conditions that, while not common, put particular pressures on those who suffer from them. Crossed eyes (strabismus) is a condition in which the two eyes do not work together; one eye or the other may turn inward, outward, upward or downward. There are different causes. But the result is poor eye control. Ophthalmologists tend to blame poor eye control on the muscles of the eye and all too frequently advise surgery. The behavioral optometrist believes differently and has a less radical, more promising approach.

The condition of strabismus occurs because the individual's vision system has not learned to make the two eyes work together as a team. In rare cases, paralyzed or partially paralyzed muscles may indeed cause lazy eye, but such paralysis occurs in a minute percentage of the population.

It is normal, during the first five or six months, for an infant's eyes to appear crossed or unaligned for brief moments while the infant is learning to use the eyes together as a team. But, if by the age of 3 1/2 months the misalignment appears to be frequent or long-lasting, or is always with the same eye, it is wise to visit a practitioner of optometric vision therapy.

Crossed eyes can also develop at a later stage, as children reach school age. Oddly enough, the development is often so gradual that parents fail to recognize it. They get used to the child's appearance and it seems normal. In this case, the problem may be noticed first by the family doctor or at school.

Crossed Eyes: A Cosmetic and Functional Problem

Two major factors are involved in crossed eyes. One, the most obvious, is appearance. Crossed eyes look funny, peculiar, different. And "different" is the last thing your school-age child wants to be. Two, because of the "difference," crossed eyes can inhibit a child's emotional and social development. They can also cause personality problems by isolating the individual from other youngsters and giving the child a poor self-image.

A child rarely outgrows crossed eyes. Therefore, parents are wise to seek help as soon as they spot the symptoms.

What Are the Choices?

For several decades, the conventional medical treatment for crossed eyes has been surgery. Today, however, the specialists in behavioral optometry strongly recommend *against surgery*, particularly in cases which are obviously vision imbalances.

The reasons are several. First, surgery usually does not offer a permanent solution to the problem. In surgery, the eye muscles are cut so that the eyes look straight (if the surgeon has judged it to the precise degree). However, since *no effort is made to teach the eyes how to work together as a team*, the underlying imbalance remains and there is a strong tendency for the eyes to turn again. In many cases, repeated operations are necessary, yet there's no guarantee of total success.

In contrast, behavioral optometric vision therapy, which opts not to use surgery or drugs, has a greater success rate in treating crossed or out-turning eyes than surgery. In fact, because it treats the underlying cause, behavioral optometry may be able to solve the problem because once the eyes learn how to work together as a team, there is less of a tendency for them to turn.

Lazy Eye, not Lazy Child

Amblyopia is often called "lazy eye" and it is a condition in which clear, sharp vision in one eye is lowered or apparently lost and cannot be improved with prescription "compensating" lenses. It affects about 2 percent of children.

The AOA tells us that there are different kinds of lazy eye. The most common type is a side effect or complication stemming from crossed eyes or from a vision condition in which one eye is much more nearsighted or farsighted than the other. In either of those situations, the two eyes send separate and different messages to the brain, which cannot integrate them. Therefore, the brain often turns off the message from one eye. Since the ability to see sharply and clearly is a learned skill, central visual acuity never develops properly in the eye that the brain has turned off.

The one-eyed vision that results can affect other vision skills, such as the ability to judge distances, although a youngster with a lazy eye will not realize this. Once again, it is left to parents and teachers to identify the condition.

Look for the child who noticeably favors one eye (head-tilting is one clue) or who has a tendency to bump into objects. Since poor vision in one eye does not necessarily mean amblyopia or lazy eye (it could be nearsightedness), amblyopia can only be definitely diagnosed by a professional examination. Remember that often the lazy-eyed child becomes one-sided in responses and movements and usually does not develop the concept of opposites; perhaps there will be difficulty in balancing and in sports. Sometimes certain activities like dancing that require using two sides of the body may be avoided.

Practitioners of optometric vision therapy believe that near- and farsightedness and astigmatism are adaptations individuals make so they can perform well. The need for such adaptations may be alleviated when the entire vision system is brought into balance.

How Behavioral Optometry Helps

Optometric vision therapy works with the visual perceptual system and the various subsystems that integrate with vision. The pathways of the vision system include neuromuscular, neurophysiological and neurosensory systems. The eyes are the external receptors for the vision system. Light, radiant energy, is converted at the retinal level into electrical energy. This energy follows the visual pathways to the visual cortex. Developmental gaps, lags, warps or distortions at any point along the way will disrupt the efficiency of the system. Optometric vision therapy is often able to :

- Prevent or modify vision imbalances such as nearsighted-ness (myopia) and astigmatism;
- Develop the visual abilities and skills needed to achieve at school, work and sports;
- Reduce or eliminate chronic health problems, including travel sickness, bed-wetting, headaches, migraines, tension, teeth-grinding, light sensitivity, muscle pain, depression, alcoholism and schizophrenia.

Computers: A Recent Threat

The video display terminal (VDT) of the modern computer is a "growing source of vision complaints," according to the Optometric Extension Program Foundation (OEP). (A nonprofit foundation, OEP has devoted many years to providing postdoctoral behavioral optometric education and publishing related papers for professionals and the general public.)

A 1985 publication reports on a variety of evidence that relates vision problems to extended use of VDTs. This evidence is drawn from studies of office workers and from a US Air Force Study of Office Automation; but with computers invading the classroom on a broader and broader scale, parents and teachers should be warned that vision problems will be encountered among children, too.

In a comparison between workers using VDTs and those who were not, the users experienced nearly double the incidence of irritated eyes, burning eyes, blurred vision and 50 percent more eyestrain. There were related physical complaints, too—headaches, aching necks, backs, shoulders and hands.

Constant computer use does produce measurable fatigue in the eye accommodation mechanism, as well as an increased blink rate. Because printed material and VDT images differ in quality, VDT characters are relatively blurred and have small area flicker. The continuous action of the eye lens may be necessary to achieve proper focus on the relatively blurred characters. The small area flicker also necessitates constant adjustment. Close range viewing of VDTs requires convergence and accommodation of the eyes for sustained periods.

Visual stress leads to lowered performance. Children react to stress by avoiding work, or work under stress with lowered-comprehension. In some cases, they adapt to stress by becoming nearsighted or suppressing the use of one eye.

Adults must be alert for the symptoms of visual problems, especially among youngsters who are now being exposed to lengthy use of computers.

5

Vision-Related Problems: Who Do You Turn to for Help?

Several kinds of doctors specialize in eye care.

The Optometrist - O.D.

The O.D. degree stands for Doctor of Optometry. It is earned after a minimum of seven years of college and graduate education. The four-year program at colleges of optometry includes biochemistry, human anatomy, endocrinology and microbiology, general pharmacology and pathology, sensory and perceptual psychology and clinic work. Optometry's areas of specialization range from contact lenses to pediatric, geriatric and sports vision. One of the most innovative is vision therapy, for which postdoctoral training is needed.

The General Optometrist - O.D.

This O.D. offers routine eye health care and refraction (the clinical measurement of the eye to determine the need for lenses). Extensive education prepares the general optometrist to detect not only ocular diseases but signs of certain health problems such as hypertension, diabetes and arteriosclerosis. Optometrists are trained to give excellent primary health care.

The Behavioral, Developmental or
Functional Optometrist -O.D.

This O.D. has postdoctoral training in optometric vision therapy . In contrast to the general optometrist and the ophthalmologist, who usually believe that visual problems stem from random or genetic biological variations, the behavioralist believes that visual problems are also triggered by environmental factors which may be developmental or induced by stress.

The Ophthalmologist - M.D.

The ophthalmologist is a medical doctor whose postdoctoral training is in diseases of the eye and eye surgery.

The Optician - This is a technician who produces and/or dispenses the optical lenses, glasses or other equipment prescribed by optometrists and ophthalmologists.

It is to the optometrist who specializes in behavioral, functional or developmental vision care that parents and teachers need to turn when—based on the symptoms described previously—they suspect a student has a vision problem.

Note: Practically speaking, parents are wise not to wait for symptoms. It is simply good health insurance to have a child's vision examined by a behavioral optometrist before age three and again before the child enters school and annually thereafter until adulthood. If this were done, we would find fewer students with learning difficulties and more adults with happier and more productive lives.

Let us repeat a warning. Checking a child's visual acuity on the time-honored Snellen eyechart, with which we are all familiar from our school days, is not enough. Nor is it enough to determine that the eyes are healthy.

The Vision Examination

A vision examination by a behavioral optometrist, particularly of a child, can be a lengthy procedure. But it is neither painful nor demanding of the patient. Properly prepared for it, a youngster can find it interesting, even fun.

A thorough examination takes from thirty to sixty minutes on the first visit and includes a battery of tests (many of which are like playing games). Specific tests given will vary with each child's individual needs. Besides the review of the child's health history and an examination to confirm the eyes' physical health, the vision examination by the behavioral optometrist includes:

- Tests of the child's ability to see sharply and clearly at near and far distances
- Tests to determine refractive status (nearsightedness, farsightedness and focusing problems)
- A check of eye coordination to be certain the eyes work as a team at both near and far distance
- A test of the ability to change focus easily from near to far and vice versa
- A check for any indication of crossed eyes or indications that the child is not using one eye
- A test of depth perception
- Motor tests to check eye-hand-foot coordination

The results of all these tests of visual functioning are then compared to an expected developmental level. Where results fall below expected levels, optometric vision therapy may be recommended.

Schools Need Thorough Vision Tests

The New York State Optometric Association (NYSOA) has designed a comprehensive vision test that can be used in schools without the help of a vision care professional. Specialists in psychology, statistics, reading and curriculum as well as pediatric optometrists collaborated in the development of the material. Sixteen independent functions of pediatric vision are checked: acuity, muscle coordination, visual motor integration, eye tracking skills, convergence, color deficiency, sensory motor coordination, fusion, stereopsis, myopia, hyperopia, astigmatism, amblyopia, binocularity and eye-hand coordination.

One of the leading manufacturers of vision therapy equipment, Bernell Corporation of South Bend, Indiana, markets the NYSOA material. Bernell, which has served the international community of vision care practitioners since the early 1950s, has devoted an entire page of its catalogs since 1986 to the NYSOA school screening battery.

By 1990, two states had enacted laws and guidelines for this type of school screening. Louisiana was the first, followed by New Jersey. In Louisiana, maverick citizen Charles Blaise was instrumental in working with lawmakers to develop Act No. 156 of the 1983 Regular Session of the Louisiana Legislature. The act directed each school system to implement a sensory screening program that includes visualization, audition and nutrition tests of schoolchildren's communication skills.

6

Vision Care:
Lenses, Therapy or Both

W hen a practitioner of optometric vision therapy examines a patient and finds evidence of a vision imbalance, different courses of action are possible: 1. lenses; 2. vision therapy procedures. When lenses and vision therapy are used together, the benefits of each are increased.

Lenses

Often, particularly when vision imbalances are minor, lenses are needed only for schoolwork (to take stress off the vision system). Behavioral optometrists base their lens prescriptions on concepts different from those used by ophthalmologists and general optometrists.

In general, the latter two groups use lenses only in one way. They prescribe "compensating" lenses, which treat symptoms not causes. For instance, if a child is nearsighted (commonly a symptom of a vision imbalance), compensating lenses can provide 20/20 eyesight. But as the imbalance worsens, as it almost always does, stronger and stronger lenses usually have to be prescribed to maintain 20/20 sight because the vision imbalance is still there.

Since this approach is sight-oriented, the underlying causes of the nearsightedness (or whatever the symptom) are not being treated. The vision system is not being brought into balance; if it were, the need for these compensating lenses might well be eliminated.

The behavioral optometrist uses lenses in various ways:

Preventive lenses—to prevent a problem in the vision system from starting in those diagnosed to be "at risk";

Developmental lenses—to support and nurture an immature vision system while helping it develop normally and help it cope with visual stress;

Remedial lenses—for a specific problem, such as an inability to sustain focusing, until that ability is adequate.

Vision Therapy

This involves an array of procedures designed to achieve or maintain an optimally balanced and flexibly functioning vision system. It aims to teach the entire vision system to operate at peak efficiency. A program tailored specifically by the behavioral optometrist to the individual patient can:

- Help prevent the development of some vision problems such as myopia;

- Aid in the proper development of vision abilities;

- Enhance the efficiency and comfort of vision functioning;

- Help cure and/or correct existing vision problems.

Good Vision Is Developed, Not Inborn

The ability to see and correctly interpret what is seen does not appear automatically at birth. It develops over a lifetime and is shaped by one's experiences and environment. Optometric vision therapy is based on the fact that vision is learned.

Some children skip steps in their vision development, sometimes because of illness. Others may not be exposed to the necessary visual experiences or learning opportunities to develop their vision skills adequately.

Modern living puts endless stresses on the vision systems of both children and adults. The impact of hours upon hours of daily TV viewing is a whole new complication, yet to be fully understood in terms of vision development. The school-age child is confronted by reading and writing and other close work repeatedly interrupted by demands to shift focus to a teacher or blackboard. An even newer potential problem is the introduction into classrooms (and offices) of the computer. Lengthy staring into a display terminal screen may cause the individual to start having difficulty focusing back and forth between text and screen. These and other stresses can start or worsen a variety of vision imbalances. Eyes may lose their ability to "team." The farsighted and nearsighted may become more so. And so on.

A program of optometric vision therapy can protect and repair the system. What the behavioral optometrist does is break down the process of vision into various components. Then the problem areas are treated by reeducating, reinforcing or developing specific vision skills such as:

- Clearness of vision at near and far distances
- Eye movement skills
- Eye focusing skills
- Eye aiming skills
- Eye-hand coordination
- Visual perception, identification and memory

You may consider that all these skills are your natural inheritance. The fact is, from infancy, they must all be enhanced through experience and learning. Most people use them well enough to get along (but often, not as well as they might). A substantial percentage of the population does not learn one or another of these skills—or, worse, is deficient in a significant number of them.

This is where optometric vision therapy comes in. The behavioral optometrist prescribes a program of visual activities which will be performed in the optometrist's office, although many are also assigned as home therapy.

The activities vary widely, depending on the individual's special needs. Some, such as walking on a balance beam or jumping on a trampoline, will seem like play to a child. Others make use of equipment that is space age in its sophistication. The repetition of these visual activities is aimed at improving vision by improving the integration of all the sensory motor activities with vision at the helm. The therapy works to enhance visual monitoring ability, visualization skills and visual perceptual abilities, among others.

Does Optometric Vision
Therapy Really Work?

This health care is structured to treat the root of vision imbalances, not just symptoms. Optometric vision therapy, according to professional organizations like the AOA, the College of Optometrists in Vision Development and the Optometric Extension Program Foundation, is a treatment program designed to teach the entire vision system to operate at peak efficiency. Based on the fact that vision is primarily a learned process that begins at birth, optometric vision therapy is used to help persons learn, relearn or reinforce specific vision skills more efficiently.

The procedures may begin by breaking bad visual habits that have developed—habits that have taught the eyes to work separately rather than together. Then they teach individuals how to use their eyes as a team, moving step by step through all the learning stages necessary to achieve normal eye teaming. (With most, Nature has already done all this, but sometimes

Nature needs a little help.) The process can take a couple of months or a year, depending on the severity of the imbalance.

Richard S. Kavner, O.D., and Lorraine Dusky wrote in their book *Total Vision* that it has been found that 75 percent of individuals with crossed eyes and 85 percent of children with vision-related learning disabilities can be helped by optometric vision therapy.

Optometrists Nathan Flax and Robert H. Duckman, in the *Journal of the American Optometric Association* for December 1978, cite a number of studies on the effects of optometric vision therapy. They cite five studies involving 439 persons who underwent optometric vision therapy for crossed eyes. Seventy-six percent attained normal two-eyed vision and 86 percent achieved straight eyes. The remainder experienced some degree of improved vision and/or straightening of the eyes.

Another study, which followed up on persons in an earlier work, confirmed that results achieved with vision therapy are long- term, not short-term. Of 81 patients who had been successfully treated for crossed eyes with vision therapy three to seven years earlier, 96 percent still had straight eyes and 89 percent had normal two-eyed vision.

Optometrists Martin H. Birnbaum, Kenneth Koslowe and Robert Sanet in the *American Journal of Optometry and Physiological Optics* for May 1977, review 23 studies involving more than 1,100 persons whose lazy eye condition was treated with vision therapy. Over 50 percent improved their visual acuity by four lines or better on the eyechart. More than 33 percent achieved 20/30 acuity or better.

The evidence is abundant. Take, for instance, our often maligned learning-disabled children. Drs. Robert M. Wold, John R. Pierce and Joan Keddington, in the *Journal of the American Optometric Association* for September 1978, find that the effectiveness of vision therapy was dramatically demonstrated in a 1978 study of 100 learning-disabled patients. Although 99 percent of them had passed a routine vision screening for eyesight, all had difficulties in one or more areas of vision. Thirty-nine percent lacked good eye-focusing skills; 96 percent could not change their eye focus easily from near to far and back; 75 percent had difficulty using their eyes together as a team; 94 percent had problems with eye movement skills; and 91 percent lacked good eye-aiming skills. After vision therapy, 80 percent had good eye-focusing skills; 75 percent could change their eye focus easily from near to far and back; 86 percent could use their eyes together as a team; 96 percent improved their eye movement skills; and 75 percent sharpened their eye-aiming skills.

Optometric Vision Therapy for Juvenile Delinquents

Studies have found that learning-related vision problems are a strong contributing factor to juvenile delinquency. Once the underlying vision problems are corrected, delinquents can be on the road to becoming productive members of society.

A seven-year federally funded study of juvenile delinquents by a team guided by Dr. Stanley Kaseno, an optometric specialist in California, showed that nearly nine out of ten youths examined had some kind of vision problem. The only approach to health care that the county had not previously involved in their treatment of these children was behavioral optometry. Lenses to fit the vision needs were prescribed and, once optometric vision training was completed, two significant changes were noted: grades improved and the reading level of the group went from 5th to 8.5 level. The figures for rearrest went from 45 percent down to 16 percent. In a 1977 Virginia study of 79 male and female juvenile delinquents with diagnosed vision-related learning disabilities, those given specific help, including vision therapy, were roughly six times less likely to come back into the court system (*Journal of Learning Disabilities*, April 1978).

Training for Athletes

Even the finest athletes, of all ages, have used optometric vision training to sharpen their skills. Quick reaction time, fast, accurate judgement of distances and objects in motion, sharp, clear images, the perception of the athlete's body attitude and its position in space related to other bodies and objects around it—all these are necessary to superior athletic performance. And they all depend on a good, balanced vision system. Behavior is reaction to information from the vision system.

One optometric study reported in the AOA *News* that even among US Olympic contenders approximately 60 percent could sharpen their competitive performance by improving their vision skills. In fact, optometric vision training played a part in helping both the US women's and men's volleyball teams to their respective bronze and gold medals in the 1984 Olympics. Many professional sports teams have learned the lesson, too, including the New York Knicks, New York Islanders, New York Yankees, Kansas City Royals, Dallas Cowboys, Chicago Black Hawks and the San Francisco 49ers among others.

A child who does poorly at sports is often simply a victim of vision problems. Since this kind of failure can affect the child's acceptance by its peers, it can warp relationships and lead to negative self-images. It may even lead to a lifetime avoidance of physical activity.

Why let it happen when help is so readily at hand?

Physical Disabilities and Low Vision

Optometric vision therapy has brought substantial improvements for those with disabilities and low vision. Dr. William V. Padula of Guilford, Connecticut, specializes in behavioral vision care for those with visual impairments, multihandicaps and traumatic brain injury. He directs the Low Vision Clinic of the Easter Seal Rehabilitation Center in New Haven,

Connecticut and is a consultant to programs for the disabled across the United States, in China and Mexico. Dr. Padula is also on the staff of the Woodmere Hospital for Traumatic Brain Injury in Connecticut. In 1988, the OEP Foundation published his *A Behavioral Vision Approach for Persons with Physical Disabilities*. This book discusses the perceptual development of visually impaired children, the needs of the visually impaired multihandicapped and brain injured and the use of optical aids for those with low vision.

Michigan, a leader in the development of comprehensive low vision programming for visually impaired children, began a Youth Low Vision Program in 1985 with state grants. Susan R. Gormezano, O.D., and Phillip Raznik, O.D., of Southfield, Michigan, are low vision specialists who have been involved in this work from the beginning. The program led to the creation of a privately funded High Vision Games, similar to special olympics, for visually impaired youngsters. Optometric vision therapy opens new horizons in the treatment of vision impairments, physical disability and traumatic injury.

Work Around the World

In the 1990s, optometric vision therapy was available in thirty-five countries. Australia, Europe, Japan, New Zealand, all have practitioners who have either visited the United States to study with American behavioral optometrists or have invited their North American colleagues to lecture abroad. Dr. Greg Gilman of Quincy, California, travelled continuously for eighteen months around the world. He gave seminars in fifty countries and an average of seventy-five people attended each seminar, although once he had an audience of 2,500 optometrists.

Dr. Glenn Swartwout of Portland, Oregon, spent two years (1983-84) in Japan, as the first director of the Optometric Center of Tokyo, which he helped to found. This center was the in-house research clinic for a major optical company, the

Sanki Optical Group. Their support and that of the Kojima family of Tokyo made the project a reality. Japan has a population roughly half that of the United States, yet the number of "refracting opticians" in Japan is the second largest in the world after America.

In 1986, the Tokyo Optical Company, Limited, the third largest optical company in Japan, invited Dr. Philip Smith of San Diego, California, a behavioral optometrist who practices sports vision, to come to Japan and share his experience with athletes in the evaluation and training of their visual skills. Dr. Smith worked with the manager and coach of the Hiroshima Carps Baseball team, winners of their division, similar to the American or National League Pennant. He also worked with a number of Japanese refracting opticians, showing them how to test and train athletes' vision skills.

Not a Magic Cure-All

A clarification here is useful. No one health therapy can help everyone. Optometric vision therapy does not help all children or adults with health, learning and behavior problems; it usually helps those whose difficulties are related to vision problems.

A wealth of reliable studies document the positive results of optometric vision therapy. If you are interested in delving more deeply into the subject, a three-part paper by Irwin Suchoff, O.D., former Dean of the College of Optometry of State University of New York, and Timothy Petito, O.D., has a definitive bibliography of such research. Part I of the Suchoff-Petito paper, "The Efficacy of Visual Therapy: Accommodative Disorders and Non-Strabismic Anomalies of Binocular Vision," published in the *Journal of the American Optometric Association* in 1986, is an invaluable reference for consumers whose insurance companies or physicians are interested in current, qualified research.

Repairing the Damage
The Team Approach

When you help youngsters with behavior or learning difficulties develop efficient vision systems, that's usually only the *first* step along the way to helping them develop fully productive lives. Frequently, these children have not developed efficient skills in reading and writing. They are behind their grade level in most studies. Good work and study habits are foreign to them. They often have mild to severe emotional problems, which may range from feelings of unworthiness to rebellious rage.

Fixing the cause of all these problems is one thing. Repairing the damage is another. Often, the repairs call for a team approach. In addition to the behavioral optometrist providing vision therapy, a team can include experts in such fields as education, psychology, nutrition and child development.

The therapy of behavioral optometry is offered in thirty-five countries around the world. In the United States, most of the fifteen colleges of optometry offer courses in vision therapy.

Many also have clinics where various types of optometric vision care are available. A number of institutions such as the SUNY College of Optometry, the Illinois College of Optometry, the Eye Institute at the Pennsylvania College of Optometry and Southern California College of Optometry place a strong emphasis on the value of teamwork. This was also the case at the internationally celebrated Gesell Institute of Human Development which was located in Connecticut for several decades.

Vision and Behavior: An Unbreakable Link

Many names stand out among the leaders of behavioral optometry. From the early pioneers such as Drs. Alexander, Brock, Getman, McCoy and Macdonald to the modern practitioners such as Drs. Apell, Flax, Francke, Forrest, Greenspan, Margach, Sherman, Solan, Streff and Wachs, their contributions have been invaluable in forging this remarkable discipline. Yet there is one individual who seems to tower over the rest: A. M. Skeffington, O.D., is generally regarded as the "father" of behavioral optometry.

In the 1920s, Skeffington began to question what could be done for vision imbalances beyond the simple prescribing of lenses to wear. His creative mind reached out beyond the boundaries of his own field of optometry to involve authorities from other disciplines as diverse as biology, physiology, psychology, neurology, physics and education. From 1928, Skeffington was the mainspring of the Optometric Extension Program for forty years. Now the Optometric Extension Program Foundation, this was the first organization to develop a wide variety of continuing education courses for its members and to publish education and information pamphlets for the public.

Arnold Gesell, M.D., for whom the Gesell Institute was named, was another of the early investigators who helped establish the foundations for this health care in the 1940s. Dr. Gesell, widely regarded as one of the world's leading pediatric psychologists and a specialist in child development, studied vision for almost a decade with a team of experts. The result was the landmark book *Vision and Its Development in Infant and Child*

. Over the decades, the critical connection between vision and behavior has been painstakingly established. Gradually, the precepts of a revolutionary new health therapy have been developed:

- Vision problems may trigger or aggravate learning or behavior problems
- Vision can be trained
- When vision is treated by optometric specialists, learning and behavior may also change and improve.

Home Vision Therapy

Many practitioners of optometric vision therapy include out-of-office or home vision therapy as part of treatment (the parents involved in such work with infants, preschool or schoolchildren often become dedicated to the therapy's concepts of prevention). However, regular office visits are important for a number of reasons. At an office, you have professionals who can analayze progress and adjust the activities where necessary. Also, the use of lenses, a critical factor in this therapy, needs to be monitored for adjustments.

The question of home procedures must always be considered carefully. Some children may need the help of an adult, but if the home situation isn't correct for that involvement, then it's wise to wait before starting work at home. Vision therapy at home for adults is often recommended but the guidelines are the same as those for youngsters.

Peripheral and binocular vision You may want to check these two vital areas. Peripheral vision, when used by both eyes simultaneously in a binocular manner, is one of the most important functions of your visual system. It lets you know where you are. It is also the foundation for the development of size, time and spatial concepts. If you know where you are when walking, balancing or running, you will not stagger or fall or bump into objects.

Check peripheral vision by standing in the middle of the room and looking straight ahead. Are you aware of all or some of the rest of the room? Ask a friend or someone in your family how much they notice of side areas when they look straight ahead. The following can help you find out the quality of your binocular peripheral vision.

The Brock String Test This device, four or five beads or buttons of different colors on a piece of string some three to four feet long, was created by Dr. Frederick Brock, one of the pioneers in the field of optometric vision therapy. It is a good example of the type of simple equipment that can be used to exercise and stimulate the vision system. When you use the Brock string, you learn a number of things:

- Are you using both eyes as a team all the time?
- Which eye is the "stronger" eye?
- What is the quality of each eye's vision?

When you focus on different beads at different times, you can develop valuable eye-teaming skills.

How to Use the Brock String Thread string through four or five beads and secure them so that they're evenly spaced one from the other. Position the first bead about twelve inches from the end of the string. Attach one end of the string at eye level to a door knob or other convenient handle (or hold it yourself) and wind the other end around your fingers. Hold the string taut, at arm's length, with the end wrapped around your finger and held against the middle of your nose; look at the bead closest to you. The Brock string can be held still or it can be rotated for focusing and teaming work. If you are using both eyes together at the same time and aiming accurately at the first bead, it will look as if there are two strings that meet in a V at the bead; the strings seem to go into the beads and come out on the other side, thus they form an X. Each string should be of equal quality, not becomefuzzy or indistinct at any place.

If the strings meet before the bead, you have a tendency to fixate or aim inaccurately or overconverge. This will cause you to hold your reading material too close, which is stressful. It might also cause you to blur at distance occasionally. If the strings meet behind the button, you are diverging.

If you see two beads side by side, you have difficulty converging. This means you probably hold your reading too far away, causing stress. Lower back problems may also result. If your eyes do not work together as a team, you rarely know this. Where there's a lack of teaming, the individual often uses first one eye then the other, at the cortical level. This results in certain behavioral characteristics. You might change your mind a great deal or have difficulty making decisions. Perhaps you have a slow response to a visual exercise such as the Brock string. This often indicates a slow starter, maybe even someone accused of being a procrastinator. The stress of hidden visual problems such as poor teaming or alternating is often the trigger for disruptive behavior.

Use the Brock string on a daily basis, if possible, if you find your binocularity is not very efficient. Don't overdo it at first if you do have problems, such as the strings meeting in front of or behind the bead at which you aim your eyes. Just as you must gradually build up endurance for physical exercise, so you must build up endurance for visual exercise. At first, spend about forty seconds on each bead, preferably at the same time each day, as many times a week as possible. Then, as you improve, you can slowly increase the time you take to do this simple but amazingly effective drill.

You have efficient binocular ability when you see two strings of the same quality. Perhaps you have learned to see the strings in the correct place but they do not stay visible clearly or steadily but flicker or fade. If so, you need to work consistently at the drill to develop efficient eye teaming that allows you to use both eyes at the same time and have consistent vision.

It's shocking to realize one doesn't always see consistently. Normally, we're not aware of vision imbalances. It's only when we start using devices like the Brock string that we begin to realize the quality of our perceptions. If you are playing sports—football, tennis, golf, baseball—you may not time your swing at the ball correctly. Analyze your own game. If you see the strings on the Brock string cross behind the bead, you sometimes swing too late. If you see the strings cross in front of the bead, you tend to swing too early.

If our vision systems are not efficient, we need to put far more effort and energy into trying to have accurate perceptions than people who have good vision. When you are driving, your brain wants to know where the road is for the left-hand turn. If you cannot see the turn of the road accurately, you will analyze the information over and over in an attempt to understand the visual input. This can be dangerous when you're behind the wheel of a car. In many situations, it can make you seem slow, even stupid.

Test Your Binocular Vision   A simple way to check if you do use both eyes at the same time can be done at home with the cardboard tube from, say, a roll of paper towel.

1. Hold the cardboard tube in one hand, position it in front of one eye and look through the tube.

2. Place your free hand, palm facing you, halfway down, at the center of the tube, by the side of the tube.

3. If you are using both eyes together, you will see a hole in your palm which matches the size of the hole that you see at the end of the tube.

4. If you are not using both eyes together, you will either look down the cardboard tube or just see your hand.

Conclusion You have efficient binocularity if you see both the tube and the hole in your palm at the same time. You are not truly binocular if you see only one or the other, if the tube and the circle are not equally distinct, or if the images blur or fade in and out. You probably knew this, if you knew you cannot view 3-D movies. What does this lack of true binocularity mean? It means that you do not have accurate depth perception. This imbalance is a drain on energy; it also leads to stress. It creates difficulties in your perception of your location and the location of objects around you. Walking, driving or sports activities become obstacle courses.

The range of home procedures is considerable. Some make use of simple objects, balls on strings, pencils, dowels; others are sophisticated. Usually, lenses are an integral part of any program. Sometimes nasal occluders (nasal or binasal tapes) are used on lenses to treat myopia, strabismus, amblyopia and suppression. Tapes of varying width are applied to spectacles to disrupt the wearer's visual habits and bring desirable changes. Practice is needed if there are to be improvements in the way individuals use their vision systems.

Warning: The Great Debate
Yet Insurance Pays and Nader Agrees

Behavioral optometry is a specialty. In the United States, it is practiced by about 12 percent of the 24,000 doctors of optometry, who have pursued the necessary extra training. On the other hand, the average ophthalmologist, family doctor, pediatrician or child psychologist usually knows little or nothing about optometric vision therapy because their education has not included courses in it. Many of them, in all good faith, condemn the idea.

In contrast, those practitioners who do know of and value the therapy have no hesitation about sharing their expertise in this matter. Allan Cott, M.D., a psychiatrist in New York City writes in *Help for Your Learning-Disabled Child* that he usually has his patients include a vision examination by a behavioral optometrist in their initial testing. He writes:

> *An examination of a learning-disabled child without a consultation and treatment by a developmental optometrist is an incomplete examination and treatment.*

Dr. Cott also points out that a child with problems grows up to become an adult with problems. Pediatrician Morris Wessel, M.D., of Cheshire, Connecticut, also discusses the value of optometric vision therapy in his book, *Raising a Healthy Child*, part of *Parents Magazine* Baby and Children series. In the foreword to Dr. Kavner's *Your Child's Vision* and in other material he has authored, as well as the book *Rickie* (about his daughter), Fredrich Flach, M.D., a New York City psychiatrist, describes optometric vision therapy as a valid, valuable health therapy. General practitioner Dorothea Linley, M.D., of Cheshire, Connecticut, suggests that material on optometric vision therapy needs to be part of "required medical reading," particularly for physicians dealing with problem children. Ophthalmologist George Dupont, M.D., of Newport Beach, California, says that he has been exposed to the optometric as well as the ophthalmological phases of eye care and that he "refers appropriate patients and in every instance they benefit a great deal."

Be warned. You will find a number of otherwise reliable advisors pooh-poohing behavioral optometry. But the large insurance companies don't. Consumer advocate Ralph Nader doesn't. Luci Johnson doesn't. A roll call of professional athletes do not. Consider the fact, also, that police across the United States apply the concepts of behavioral optometry daily in sobriety tests of drivers.

How US Police Use the Therapy's Concepts

Since 1970, the Connecticut State Police have used the behavioral optometric vision programs Dr. Forkiotis developed for them. A consultant for the US Department of

Transportation Research Office and the National Health Traffic Safety Administration for drug-testing detection and the National Standardized Behavioral Sobriety tests, Dr. Forkiotis has presented expert witness courses to police training officers, state prosecuting attorneys and county attorneys around America since the 1980s.

The scientific basis for standardized behavioral sobriety tests in the US (alcohol gaze nystagmus) is based on the concepts of behavioral optometry. The police tests involve vision and the vision system and are used as field tests to determine whether drivers are under the influence of alcohol or drugs. Until the development of this testing, such cases had often been thrown out of court for lack of evidence. In 1985, the use of such tests was supported in a landmark US court decision. Experts such as Dr. Forkiotis help US police learn to test suspicious drivers for nystagmoid oscillation, the uncontrolled, erratic eye movement that develops when alcohol or drugs are in one's body.

What does all this prove? Major health insurance companies such as Aetna and Blue Cross/Blue Shield pay only for health care that they have investigated and found sound and necessary. Their coverage includes optometric vision care.

Ralph Nader does not lightly endorse *anything*. But in 1980, this redoubtable guardian of consumer interest endorsed optometric vision therapy in the strongest terms.

Of many examples, one will suffice: an article on optometric vision care in the *Wall Street Journal* of May 29, 1985, quoted Aetna Life & Casualty Company: "We're convinced of its value." The company added that they have offered coverage for optometric vision therapy for "at least a decade." Why? Indisputable evidence has established its value.

Look at the back of this handbook for a selection of the reputable scientific studies that led Aetna Life (and other insurance companies) to such a decision; note the professional journals which published them. You'll also find titles of some of the many pamphlets published by the various professional organizations. A well-documented consumer's guide to the therapy is the book *Suddenly Successful, How Behavioral Optometry Helps You Overcome Learning, Health and Behavior Problems* by the coauthors of this handbook.

So don't be dissuaded by an advisor who has not looked as deeply into the question of optometric vision therapy as Aetna. Or Nader.

9

A Home Guide for Infant Vision Development

Most babies are born with healthy eyes, free from disease and vision problems. Learning to *use* these eyes is one of the critical first steps in a newborn's development.

Since infants spend a large part of their time learning to see, parents of new babies will be glad to read there's a lot they can do to help infants develop healthy vision systems.

Whether it's the presence of bright wallpaper, the frequent repositioning of the crib or a colorful mobile to provide variety and movement, the points are simple and effective. Our source is the American Optometric Association's background paper on infants' vision and the guidelines developed over many years by the Infants' Vision Clinic at SUNY in New York City, under the direction of Elliott Forrest, O.D.

Early Visual Stimulation

Keep a dim light burning in the nursery at night so the infant will have something to look at on awakening.

Move the crib regularly, as well as the baby's position in the crib so that light will stimulate each eye. It's preferable to use clear bumper guards so vision is not obstructed.

Approach, change, feed and even play with the baby from different positions. Talk to your baby as you move around the room; this gives the infant a moving object to follow. During the day, place the child in different rooms so that new sights, objects, patterns and different light will stimulate the vision system.

For the first two months, keep a bright mobile dangling outside the crib to provide variety and movement. At about eight weeks, move the mobile over the crib so the baby can touch it. This permits reinforcement of tactual and visual information.

Hand-Eye Coordination

Play peek-a-boo and play patty-cake.

Provide blocks, rattles, balls and other toys for the baby to touch, bang and throw. Use objects large enough so they can't be swallowed. As the child gets older, make available toys (including pots and pans) to stack, nest, build, string, toss, push, pull, pound, take apart and put together. Clay or play dough, puzzles, tracing and coloring are also good.

General Visual-Motor Coordination

Give the child freedom to explore. Avoid the restraints of a playpen, crib and high chair when they are not required. Let the child move around as much as possible.

Encourage the child to wiggle, roll, crawl and creep. This helps coordinate the two sides of the body efficiently, an ability that is reflected in the coordination of the two eyes.

Parents, therefore, should not encourage their babies to walk before the crawling and creeping phases. Set up an obstacle course of boxes, chairs and tables so that the child can creep under, over and between objects.

When the child can walk, encourage the use of a wheelbarrow or some other push-and-balance toy. Encourage the child to run, jump, balance, hop and climb.

Match Vision With Other Sensory Motor Systems

Whenever possible, talk and play with the child. Tell stories and sing songs together.

Offer different objects and have the child tell which is heavier, lighter or noisier when dropped.

These are some of the ways you can help get your child's vision system off to a healthy start. It cannot be repeated often enough: the child has to learn to see. We are not born with sophisticated visual abilities.

Adults can depend on vision alone to discriminate and understand the size, shape, texture and weight of objects. Infants need help to understand this type of information. They are dependent in the learning process on touching, feeling, squeezing—tactile evidence that allows them to confirm what their vision notes.

As children grow, they will start to base their judgments of texture, shape, size and weight of objects on visual assessment alone. The sight of a ball will trigger their memories of how it feels and what it weighs without the need for tactile evidence that was necessary earlier.

But in the early stages, the infant's vision system must be carefully nurtured for balanced development.

Infant Vision Needs Examination, Too

Perhaps the most important safeguard recommended by the AOA is that unless signs of problems occur earlier, a child's first thorough vision examination needs to be given by the time your child is three years old. The doctor of optometry who specializes in behavioral, developmental or functional optometry is best qualified to handle this examination.

This examination will cover more than simply determining that the child's eyes are healthy, with the ability to rate well, even as high as 20/20 on the eye chart. It will examine the total vision system to make sure that it is in balance and functioning efficiently and at the appropriate level for a three-year-old. The examination should be repeated again before the youngster enters school and annually thereafter until adulthood.

10

How to Find Help

If you are looking for a doctor of behavioral optometry in your area, the most direct source of information might well be your local general optometrist, who can usually give you the name of a colleague who specializes in behavioral vision care. You can also contact either the College of Optometrists in Vision Development or the Optometric Extension Program Foundation or the colleges of optometry in the United States. Other groups include the European Society of Optometrists and the Australasian College of Behavioural Optometry. Addresses are all in the next few pages.

If you have a child who has learning or behavior problems and hasn't yet had a behavioral optometric vision examination, why not have one done promptly? It might well reveal a vision imbalance that has been missed by conventional optometric and ophthalmological examinations and which could be corrected with the proper treatment.

Don't hesitate to phone to discuss your needs. Ask how long an examination usually takes. You cannot have a thorough behavioral vision examination in less than thirty minutes; often it takes forty-five to sixty minutes. Dr. Richard Apell, when director of Gesell's Department of Vision, said that at the Institute they often needed up to ninety minutes because many of the patients had severe learning problems and more than twenty visual skills vital to learning need to be tested. Make sure you receive a "yes" answer to each of the following questions before you make an appointment.

1. Do you give a full series of nearpoint vision tests?

2. Do you give work- or school-related visual perception tests?

3. Do you provide full vision care and visual training in your office or will you refer me to a colleague if needed?

College Clincs

Many of the fifteen colleges of optometry in the United States and many of those in the thirty-five countries around the world where this therapy is practiced have clinics that offer various types of vision care. Most also have faculty who have private practices. Be sure to ask for the names of those who practice behavioral, functional or developmental optometric vision care.

A number of centers offer behavioral optometric and psycho-educational diagnoses and therapy geared either to slow learners or the learning disabled. Among these in the United States are the Learning & Development Center in Philadelphia, Pennsylvania, of which Martin Kane, O.D., is director, and the Learning Center, directed by Al Sutton, O.D., in Miami Beach, Florida. Harry Wachs, O.D., who specializes in a Piagetian approach to learning-related problems, is Director of the Reading Center, George Washington University, Washington, D.C.

There have also been a variety of research projects, some involving school systems. One, initially sponsored by OEPF, was directed by John Streff, O.D., of the NOEL Center, Lancaster, Ohio. The Gesell Institute had another in the Connecticut school system.

If you have difficulty finding addresses for clinics, centers or practitioners, one of the professional groups whose names and addresses follow may be able to help, but double-check that the optometrists actually practice behavioral, developmental or functional optometry vision therapy by asking questions like those previously mentioned.

Professional Organizations

The American Academy of Optometry was founded in 1922 with the express purpose of fostering the continued advancement of the education and knowledge of practicing optometrists. The academy publishes a monthly journal, the *American Journal of Optometry and Physiological Optics.* In addition, it publishes educational articles and textbooks. The academy holds annual educational forums, offers postgraduate courses and encourages research and scientific investigations in optometry and related fields.

The American Academy of Optometry
Attn: Chairman of the Diplomate in
Binocular Vision & Perception
118 North Oak St.
Owatonna, MN 55060

The American Optometric Association (AOA) represents more than 24,000 doctors of optometry and students of optometry in the United States. Founded in 1898, the AOA is a federation of local associations representing zones, states and the District of Columbia. A majority of practicing optometrists in the United States are members. The AOA publishes The *Journal of the American Optometric Association, AOA News* and a helpful selection of informative booklets for consumers and writers. AOA publications cover a broad spectrum of optometry, from material on the nurturing of infants' vision to advice on contact lenses.

The American Optometric Association
Communications Division
243 North Lindbergh Blvd.
St. Louis, MO 63141

The Australasian College of Behavioural Optometrists is an international, nonprofit organization that provides continuing education and research in vision. The college was founded in 1988 from a membership that had worked for decades in association with the OEP Foundation of America. The college publishes a quarterly journal, *Behavioural Optometry*

The Australasian College of Behavioural Optometrists
Suite B, 233 MacQuarie St.
Liverpool, N.S.W.,
AUSTRALIA 2170

The European Society of Optometrists is a nonprofit organization dedicated to promoting the education of behavioral optometry throughout Europe. The society was founded in 1967 and its quarterly journal, *Communication*, is published in six languages.

The European Society of Optometrists
P.O. Box 569, Bruxelles, 1
B-1000 Bruxelles; BELGIUM

The Optometric Extension Program Foundation (OEPF) is international in scope. Founded in 1928, it is the principal provider of postgraduate education to optometrists and was the first organization to develop a wide variety of continuing education courses for optometrists and to publish pamphlets for the general consumer. OEPF also publishes the *Journal of Behavioral Optometry*. These are some of their most popular publications:

When a Bright Child Has Trouble Reading: Learning Problems ;

Learning Lenses in Beginning Grades: Stress-relieving Lenses;

Psychological Effects of Visual Training;

It's Never Too Late to Treat a Lazy Eye.

Optometric Extension Program Foundation
2912 South Daimler St.
Santa Ana, CA 92705-5811

Many of the books recommended in this book may be ordered from the OEP's *VisionExtension, Inc.*, which provides supplies and materials to behavioral optometrists. VisionExtension, Inc., sponsors seminars and has a comprehensive catalog of its patient information publications, video and audio tapes, computer software and vision therapy equipment. For information contact:

VisionExtension, Inc.
2912 South Daimler St., Ste. 100
Santa Ana, CA 92705-5811

The College of Optometrists in Vision Development (COVD) is a certifying body for practitioners of comprehensive vision care. Now an international organization, COVD was created in 1970 by a merger of other behavioral optometric groups around the US.

The COVD works with other professional organizations such as the AOA, the OEPF and the American Optometric Student Association, among the many concerned with providing maximum care for the public. They cooperate with the National Association for Children With Learning Disabilities, government agencies and with many non-optometric groups who are interested in related problems.

COVD publishes the *Journal of Optometric Vision Development* and educational pamphlets for optometrists, professionals in health care, parents and educators.

The College of Optometrists in Vision Development
P.O. Box 285
Chula Vista, CA 92010

The Connecticut Society for the Preservation of Vision (CSPV) was founded in March 1983 by parents whose children had visual dysfunctions that had not been identified as the underlying cause of learning differences and problems in school. A nonprofit group staffed by volunteers, its activities were initially funded by grants. It aims to bring the public information about behavioral optometry and vision therapy. These goals are in their bylaws:

1. Identify the visually disadvantaged perso;.

2. Disseminate information on the importance of vision and options for proper care;

3. Encourage and support research in vision;

4. Provide resources and support to persons involved with visual welfare.

The society holds informational meetings and will send members to speak to groups wishing to learn about optometry vision care. They go behond these basics. CSPV offers public servies that include instructional workshops and seminars, public meetings, parent support and advocate service in schools, a library information center and screenings, which are basic vision analyses for individuals or groups. They also train volunteers to handle comprehensive vision screenings. A complete screening includes evaluation, interpretation, consultations and recommendations, with follow-up consultations with schools or other professionals as needed. Founder members Linda de Francesco, Shirley Brog Kondo, Margie L. Rosenberg and Henry E. Rosenberg were themselves trained by Drs. Forkiotis, Padula and Quinones of Connecticut.

As an example of how the vision screenings of CSPV are used, the society was invited to the remedial learning center at the University of New Haven for several consecutive years to give vision screenings for several hundred students. Not surprisingly, a high number of the students examined by the society had vision imbalances. Regretfully, the follow-through in such a situation is far from complete. Youngsters in remedial education often do not find it easy to initiate or cope with office appointments for optometric vision therapy or home procedures. Even something which seems simple, wearing the lenses, may be really difficult for these youngsters. The society's legacy to the university was to train four instructors in vision screening methods.

The society has written a training manual specifically for the nonprofessional. CSPV also has developed a screening course which is available upon request. The course is about ten hours long, with five sessions, each lasting about two hours. Practice sessions are needed and review courses are offered. The group created screening procedures for the Headstart program in New Haven. In fact, in the spring of 1985, they screened 150 Headstart preschoolers.

CSPV's parent advocate offers support and assistance to parents of learning-different children. The process helps to lessen the gap between the doctor's office and the school and usually results in a good resolution of the child's problems.

"So many parents called to say that their children were having trouble. Although often the schools had given testing, help was needed to plan for and obtain the appropriate services to fit the needs of the children," the society explains. One of their founder members has specific training with Connecticut Public Law 94-142, which is used as the basis for determining the rights of parents.

The society's goals are to continue its efforts to bring information to consumers as well as to train more volunteers to become vision screeners. It offers vision screenings whenever possible, at businesses, educational institutions, health fairs, even private homes—wherever requests take them. Write for information if you are interested in helping establish a similar organization in your community.

Connecticut Society for the Preservation of Vision
P.O. Box 7355
New Haven, CT 06519

Volunteers for Vision, Inc. is a Texas-based organization created in 1965 under the Community Action Program and Project Head Start. Its purpose is to instruct volunteers on how to conduct screening programs for three- to six-year-olds. These programs may be at preschool centers, parochial schools, public schools or federally sponsored day care centers, wherever there is concern for the visual welfare of children. The screening programs are never a substitute for the complete visual examination that can be made only by a professional in the field of vision care, but Volunteers for Vision, Inc. offers a valuable service which has helped many. Their booklet, the *Manual of Instructions, A Guide for the Vision Screening of Children,* is available at no cost and the organization's secretary is glad to discuss with educational institutions how a screening program can be developed.

Volunteers for Vision, Inc.
P.O. Box 2211
Austin, TX 78768

Parents Active for Vision Education (PAVE) was founded in 1988 in San Diego, California. The president, Marjie Thompson, the parent of a child whose life was changed by vision therapy, has worked as a therapist since 1979 in the Lemon Grove, California, practice of optometrists Sanet, Hillier and Treganza. She gathered together other parents whose children had also suffered the effects of undetected performance-related vision problems to form the organization.

PAVE's purpose is to "raise awareness among children, parents, educators and the medical community of the critical relationship between vision and achievement." PAVE wants all children tested for the four Fs (focusing, fusion, fixation and form perception) before being taught the three Rs. The group promotes and coordinates comprehensive performance-related school vision screenings. They arrange lectures on vision and learning, stress-relieving vision hygiene and how to structure the home and classroom for maximum visual learning. PAVE sponsored the first comprehensive vision education program in a San Diego school. PAVE's monthly educational meetings are well attended and they are successful in their efforts to share news of the benefits of optometric vision therapy with parents, educators, psychologists, pediatricians and other professionals. If you are interested in establishing a PAVE chapter in your community contact:

Parents Active for Vision Education
National Headquarters
7331 Hamiel Avenue
San Diego, CA 92120

Recommended Reading and Viewing

The general reader doesn't have a wide choice of books about behavioral optometry. Arnold Gesell's volume, *Vision— Its Development in Infant* and Child, is the fruit of almost a decade of intensive work by a team of experts. It paved the way for probing research into the connection between behavior and vision by the Gesell Institute's Department of Vision. Clearly written, it is aimed at professionals in the fields of psychology, optometry and education. First published in 1940, *Vision* does not have any information on the subsequent development and practice of behavioral optometry; nevertheless, it is an illuminating introduction to the origins of behavioral optometry.

In contrast, *Total Vision* and *Your Child's Vision* by Richard Kavner, O.D. (the former with Lorraine Dusky), are exceptionally fine books for general readers with a wealth of information on vision and optometric vision therapy.

Two books by Etta V. Rowley offer a valuable approach to vision care for general readers. *Enhance Your Child's Development* traces movement patterns from birth to walking age. It encourages parents to enhance their infant's development by using movement. The activities suggested are planned so that they help develop the correct foundation for efficient vision. *Integrating Mind, Brain and Body through Movement* is a manual of over fifty activities that help balance and body rhythm. The goals and benefits of each activity are explained.

Dr. Stephen Miller authored *The Eye Care Book for Computer Users.* A practical guide to productive and comfortable work at the computer, this book is easy to read. It explains factors that can produce visual stress in the workplace and discusses how to reduce or avoid such problems.

Helpful Periodicals

The professional journals such as the *Journal of Behavioral Optometry*, the *Journal of the American Optometric Association, American Journal of Optometry and Physiological Optics* and the *Journal of Learning Disabilities* all have excellent articles. Your optometrist may have copies which you can borrow, or ask your library for an interlibrary loan, if possible, from one of the colleges of optometry.

The American Optometry Association publishes good material, particularly the *Optometric Care Advice for Infants and Children, News Backgrounder* and *Vision Therapy News Backgrounder*, and OEPF publishes many pamphlets, such as "Spelling: A Visual Skill" and those listed previously. All are concise yet informative. You'll find addresses in the previous section dealing with these organizations. If buying in quantity, you can ask for group rates.

Videos

Several tapes are available from OEPF: *All Children Learn Differently*, which was developed by the Association for Children with Learning Disabilities (Orange County Chapter), is a thirty-minute VHS video narrated by Steve Allen. It is ideal for parents or small groups ($49.95).

Vision and Learning (VHS), by Dr. Sharon Luckhardt, also available from OEPF, demonstrates signs and symptoms of learning-related visual problems and is designed for educators and parents. It runs for nine and a 1/2 minutes and costs $35.00.

The Bernell Corporation offers *Your Eyes and Video Display Terminals*, prepared in association with Dr. C. Shearer. This VHS tape offers solutions to problems associated with today's computer-designed offices and includes material on vision and the association with lighting, ergonomics and multifocal lens applications in actual office environments. Twenty minutes long, the cost is $85.00

Books

Dawkins, H. R., Edelman, E. & Forkiotis, C. *Suddenly successful.* Santa Ana, Calif., VisionExtension, Inc. 1991.

Friedman, E. & Lulow, K. Dr. *Friedman's vision training program.* New York, N.Y., Bantam Books, 1983.

Gesell, A. et al. *Vision—its development in infant and child.* New York, N.Y., Harper & Row, 1971 (1st Edition 1940). Available through VisionExtension, Inc., Santa Ana, Calif.

Getman, G. N. *How to develop your child's intelligence.* Irvine, Calif. Research Publications, 1982 (Orig. pub. 1958). Available through VisionExtension, Inc. Santa Ana, Calif.

Gregory, R. L. *Eye and brain.* New York World University Library:McGraw-Hill, 1966.

Hoopes, A. & Hoopes, T. *Eye power*. New York, N.Y., Knopf, 1979.

Kavner, R. & Dusky L. *Total vision*. New York, N.Y., A & W. Publishers, 1979. Available through VisionExtension, Inc., Santa Ana, Calif.

Kavner, R. *Your child's vision*. a parent's guide to seeing, growing, and developing. New York, N.Y., Simon & Schuster, Inc., 1985. Available through VisionExtension, Inc., Santa Ana, Calif.

Miller, S. *Eye care book for computer users*. Available through VisionExtension, Inc., Santa Ana, Calif.

Rowley, E. V. *Enhance your child's development*. Available through VisionExtension, Inc., Santa Ana, Calif.

Rowley, E. V. *Integrating mind, brain and body through movement*. Available through VisionExtension, Inc., Santa Ana, Calif.

Seiderman A. & Schneider S.*The Athletic Eye*. Hearst, New York, N.Y., 1983

Solan, H. A., ed. *The treatment and management of children with learning disabilities*. Springfield, Ill., Charles C. Thomas, 1982.

Streff, J., Ames, A. B., Gillespie, J. *Stop school failure*. New York, N.Y., Harper & Row, 1972.

Appendixes
American Colleges of Optometry (by state)

University of Alabama
  School of Optometry,
  The Medical Center
University Station
Birmingham, AL 35294

University of California Berkeley
  School of Optometry
360 Minor Hall
Berkeley, CA 94720

Southern California College of
  Optometry
2575 Yorba Linda Blvd.
Fullerton, CA 92631-1699

Illinois College of Optometry
3241 South Michigan Avenue
Chicago, IL 60616

Indiana University School of
  Optometry
800 East Atwater Avenue
Bloomington, IN 47401

New England College of
  Optometry
424 Beacon Street
Boston, MA 02115

Ferris State College of
  Optometry
Big Rapids, MI 49307

University of Missouri, at
  St. Louis, School of Optometry
8001 Natural Bridge Road
St. Louis, MO 63121

The Ohio State University
  College of Optometry
8 West 10th Street
Columbus, OH 43210

The College of Optometry
  Pacific University
2043 College Way
Forest Grove, OR 97116

Pennsylvania College of
  Optometry
1200 West Godfrey Avenue
Philadelphia, PA 19141

Inter-American University of
  Puerto Rico
  School of Optometry
G.P.O. Box 3255
San Juan, PR 00936

State University of New York
  State College of Optometry
122 East 25th Street
New York, NY 10010

Southern College of Optometry
1245 Madison Avenue
Memphis, TN 38104

University of Houston
  College of Optometry
4901 Calhoun
Houston, TX 77004

Scientific Studies

This small selection is from a wealth of reputable scientific studies which establish the efficiency of behavioral optometric vision care. A full bibliography is in "The Efficacy of Visual Therapy: Accommodative Disorders and Non-Strabismic Anomalies of Binocular Vision," Part I of III, by Drs. I. Suchoff and G. T. Petito, in the *Journal of the American Optometric Association*, 1986. Scientific studies are reviewed in the professional journals listed in "Helpful Periodicals." *The Journal of the College of Vision Development* and OEP Foundation also publish bibliographies of studies.

Bachara, G. H., and Zaba, J. N. "Learning Disabilities and Juvenile Delinquency: Beyond the Correlation." *J. Learning Disabilities* 2 (4), April 1978.

Birnbaum, M., Koslow, K., Sanet R. "Success in amblyopia therapy as a function of age: a literature review." *Am. J. Optom. & Physiol. Opt.* 54 (4):269-275, 1977.

Ciuffreda, K. J., Kenyon, R. V., Stark, L. "Different rates of functional recovery of eye movements during orthoptic treatment in an adult amblyope. *Invest. Opthal. & Vis. Sci.* 18 (2):213-219, 1979.

Ciuffreda, K. J., Goldrich, S. G., Neary, C. "Use of eye movement auditory biofeedback in the control of nystagmus," *Am. J. Optom. & Physiol. Opt.* 59 (5):396-409, 1982.

Cooper, J., Selenow, A., Ciuffreda, K. J., Feldman, J., Faverty, J., Hokoda, S., Silver, J. "Reduction of aesthenopia in patients with convergence insufficiency after fusional vergence training." *Am. J. Optom & Physiol. Opt.* 60 (12):982-989, 1983.

Daum, K. "The course and effect of visual training on the vergence system." *Am. J. Optom. & Physiol. Opt.* 59 (3):223-227, 1982.

Daum, K. "Accommodative insufficiency." *Am. J. Optom. & Physiol. Opt.* 60 (5):352-359, 1983.

Flax, N., Duckman, R. "Orthoptic treatment of strabismus." *J. Amer. Optom. Assoc.* 49 (12):1353-1360, 1978.

Goldrich, S. "Optometric therapy of divergence excess strabismus." *Am. J. Optom. & Physiol. Optics.* 57 (1):7-14, 1980.

Goldrich, S. "Oculomotor biofeedback therapy for exotropia." *Am. J. Optom. & Physiol. Optics.* 59 (4):306-317, 1982.

Hoffman, L., Cohen, A., Feur, G., Klayman, L. "Effectiveness of optometric therapy for strabismus in a private practice." *Am. J. Optom. & Physiol. Opt.* 47 (12):990-995, 1970.

Ludiam, W., Kleinman, B. "The long range results of orthoptic treatment of strabismus." *Am. J. Optom. & Physiol. Opt.* 42 (11):647-684, 1965.

Peters, H. B. "Vision Care of Children in a Comprehensive Health Program." *J. Am. Opt. Assn.* 37 (12), December 1966, updated statistics to 1979.

Selenow, A., Ciuffreda, K. "Vision function recovery during orthoptic therapy in an exotropic amblyope with high unilateral myopia." *Am. J. Optom. & Physiol Opt.* 60 (8):659-666, 1983.

Solan, H. "A Rationale for the Optometric Treatment and Management of Children with Learning Disabilities." *J. Learning Disabilities.* 14 (10), December 1981.

Solan, H., Mozlin, R., Rumpf, D. "The Relationship of Perceptual- Motor Development to Learning Readiness in Kindergarten: A Multivariate Analysis." *J. Learning Disabilities.* 18 (6), June/July 1985.

Vaegan: "Convergence and divergence show longer and sustained improvements after short isometric exercises." *Am. J. Optom. & Physiol. Opt.* 56 (1):22-33, 1979.

Weisz, C. L. "Clinical therapy for accommodative responses: transfer effects on performance." *J. Am. Optom. Assoc.* 50 (2):209-214, 1979.

Index

Accommodation, 12, 22
Acuity, visual, 11, 16, 20, 25, 26, 32
Adults, 13, 39
Alcoholism, 8, 21
Alexander, E. B., 38
Amblyopia, 20
American Academy of Optometry, 53
American Journal of Optometry and Physiological Optics, 32, 53
AOA News, 34
American Optometric Association, 1, 15, 20, 31, 47, 53
Apell, R., 38,
Arteriosclerosis, ix, 24
Astigmatism, 17, 18, 21, 26
Athletes, 34, 35

Behavior, 10, 11, 39
Behavioral optometry, see Optometry Bernell Corp., 26
Binocularity, 12, 20, 26, 39, 40, 42, 43
Birnbaum, M., 32
Blaise, C., 26
Blepharitis, 15
Brock, F., 38
Brock string, 40

Children, preschool, 14
China, 35
College of Optometrists in Vision Development, vi, 31, 51
Computer use, 15, 16, 21, 29

Connecticut Society for the Preservation of Vision, 56
Convergence, 2, 12, 41
Coordination, eye-hand, 13
Cornea, 17
Cott, A., 43, 44

Delinquent, juvenile, 1, 2, 5, 33
Depression, 8, 21
Diabetes, viii, 24
Disablity learning, 2, 8, 36, 37, 39
  physical, 34
Divergence, 12
DuPont, G., 44
Driving Under the Influence, 45
Dyslexic, 2, 5

Easter Seal Rehabilitation Center, 34
Edelman, E., i
Eye, 21
  crossed or turned, 9, 12,18-20, 25, 32
  disease, 15, 47
  exam, 17, 25, 50
  lazy, 18, 20, 32
  tracking, 26

Farsight, 3, 12, 14, 17, 21, 25
Fixation, 2, 12
Flach, F., 6-7, 44
Flax, N., v, 38
Focus and focusing, vii, 12, 17-18, 25, 29, 33, 40
Forrest, E., v, 38, 47
Forkiotis, C., v, 45, 56

Reviews of *The Suddenly Successful Student*

"Despite years of continuous success in aiding children and adults with visually related learning and performance problems, many parents and teachers are still unaware of the magnitude of optometric contributions to this important area. This book attempts to fill this gap."

> Elliott B. Forrest, O.D., Infants' Vision Clinic,
> College of Optometry, State University of New York.

"At last, a handbook for the general reader, and it's good enough to recommend for my courses."

> Charles B. Margach, O.D., Professor of Optometry,
> Southern California College of Optometry.

"...aimed at the general public...succeeds admirably, discussing the history and background of optometric vision training...."

> Martin H. Birnbaum, O.D., New York

"...relevant (and revelatory) to health professionals and general readers. A must for all libraries, it has the potential to help many."

> Tom Rose, O.D., Ohio, President,
> College of Optometrists in Vision Development.

"A readable and thorough presentation of visual dysfunction which often results in significant learning difficulties and behavioral problems in children, adolescents and adults."

> Morris Wessel, M.D., Pediatrician,
> Clinical Professor of pediatrics,
> Yale-New Haven, Connecticut.

"I learned a lot. Even general practitioners need to know the applications of optometric vision therapy to avoid prolonging patients' problems."

> Dorothea Linley, M.D., General Practitioner,
> Connecticut.

About The Authors

Hazel Richmond Dawkins is a veteran editor-writer whose career began in London's Fleet Street newspaper world and has since taken her to Paris, Geneva and New York City. She has worked for major publishers including Harper & Row and Columbia University Press.

Ellis S. Edelman, O.D., received his Doctorate in Optometry from the Pennsylvania College of Optometry and is a graduate of the Gesell Institute's postdoctoral course in behavioral optometry. An Associate of the College of Vision Development and the Optometric Extension Program Foundation, Dr. Edelman specializes in optometric vision care at Newtown Square, Pennsylvania.

Constantine Forkiotis, O.D., was a classmate of Dr. Edelman at both the Pennsylvania College of Optometry and the Gesell Institute. A Fellow of the American Academy of Optometry and the College of Vision Development, Dr. Forkiotis is active in many organizations, including the Connecticut State Board of Education. In private practice, Dr. Forkiotis specializes in optometric vision care in Fairfield, Connecticut.

The Connecticut State Police have used the behavioral optometric vision programs Dr. Forkiotis developed for them since 1970. A consultant for the US Department of Transportation Research Office and the National Health Traffic Safety Administration for drug-testing detection and the National Standardized Behavioral Sobriety tests, Dr. Forkiotis was invited by the State of Iowa to present an expert witness course to police training officers, state prosecuting attorneys, county attorneys and behavioral optometrists in 1985.
